IN HER STEPS

MEMOIRS OF THREE YEARS SPENT AT
THE JOHN SEALY COLLEGE OF NURSING
UNIVERSITY OF TEXAS
GALVESTON, TEXAS
1941-1944

DEDICATED
TO THE MEMORY OF
FLORENCE NIGHTINGALE

BY

ELLEN BEATRICE FRANKE RICHTER

Poetry Publications
By
Ellen Beatrice Franke Richter

LAMENTATIONS OF A SMALL INVESTOR
REFLECTIONS OF A SMALL INVESTOR
BARNEY
THE GATHERING PLACE

Prose Publications
By
Ellen Beatrice Franke Richter

GROUP NURSING
AN EVER WIDENING CIRCLE
IN HER STEPS

223 Pilgrim Dr.
San Antonio, TX 78313
(210)-342-0628

ISBN: 0692566627
ISBN-13: 978-0692566626

Red Flannel Quilt Publishing
Bellville, TX 77418

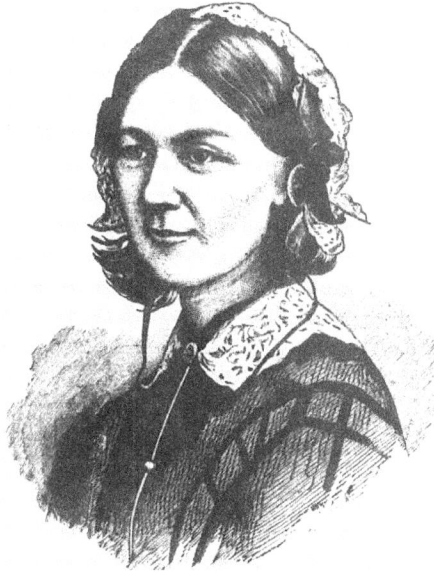

Portrait of Florence Nightingale
Australian Town and Country Journal, Published: 1875

DEDICATION

Florence Nightingale (1820-1910) is credited with bringing the Nursing Care of patients into the "modern times." Miss Nightingale was a driving force "who raised nursing to a respectable profession for women and whose far-sighted reforms have influenced the nature of modern health care." In her NOTES ON NURSING written in 1860 she laid down "the principles of nursing: careful observation and sensitivity to the patient's needs."

Quotes credit: from "Florence Nightingale" an article from the Florence Nightingale Museum website in London, England.

TABLE OF CONTENTS

Photo Credits: All photos are from the author's family picture albums, except the ranch house as noted. The cover is a colored woodcut from 1855, depicting Florence Nightingale in the Barrack hospital in Scutari, Albania, at the time of the Crimean War. A photo of Bea in her nursing uniform from 1944 is superimposed.

ACKNOWLEDGMENTS

First, I wish to recognize our instructors at the John Sealy College of Nursing in Galveston, Texas who taught us the Art of Nursing while following the precepts of Florence Nightingale. These instructors were dedicated to and meticulous in the teaching of good patient care. This program was a three year diploma program to prepare each student to become a Registered Nurse. We received clinical experience in all the patient areas in the hospital. Because of the large number of available areas for clinical practice the Nursing Program at the John Sealy Hospital was considered one of the best in the State of Texas in 1941, if not the best.

Second, let me point out the constant presence of change in our lives. During the years of 1941-1944 two memorable changes occurred. Penicillin, a fabulous new medication, came into use for patients. Also, World War II began which turned our way of living upside down.

Third, we do not go through Life alone. Many people help us along our way. Here, I would like to give thanks to Doris Walters Franke who has helped me format this memoir. Her help and support have been essential in the completion of this visit to the past.

Now, I invite you to join me on a return trip to how life was lived in a pre-plastic, pre-landfills, pre-credit card, pre-TV, pre-internet, pre-iPhone 1941 world. That time existed and I was there! We, too, were rushing towards tomorrow as we dealt with our present. So let us turn the page and see what the yesteryear of 1941 was like and get a glimpse of patient care as it was practiced then.

PROLOGUE

Where do you start when you have a story to tell? How do you find the beginning? The memories providing substance to this story are intertwined like a jumbled up bunch of string. There is a beginning somewhere if I can only find it. More complicated after I find what I think is the beginning I discover some tantalizing bit that should go before it, and wouldn't it be fun to include it in the tale. What to leave out is as difficult as what to put in. After searching for the beginning of this tale I have decided it is best just to start.

On starting I found, much to my surprise, the beginning of this story is in April of 1820 when Florence Nightingale was born while her parents were visiting in Florence, Italy. I had intended to start this tale in September of 1941 only to find the past casts long shadows into the present. The past in nursing and the improvement of hospitals rests firmly upon the endeavors of this English lady who came from a wealthy family with influential friends who helped her in her later endeavors. Florence Nightingale's father tutored her in foreign languages, math and science. At seventeen she had "a calling by God" but did not know in what direction the calling would take her. She was an adept student with definite wishes of her own. Her life continued through a visit to Rome with friends and a visit to Kaiserwerth, a hospital and school for deaconesses, near Dusseldorf.

After returning to England, with her parent's permission she went to Kaiserwerth in 1850 and took a three month nursing course. After becoming Superintendent of the Establishment for Gentlewomen During Illness at #1 Harley Street, London, her friend Sidney Herbert, Minister of War, appointed her to take nurses to Scutari in 1854 during the Crimean War. There in the barracks hospital she saw the need for sanitation in order to make the place habitable and healthy for the soldiers housed there. After a two year stay she returned to England and there concerned herself with reforming the Army Medical Services. In 1860 she established the Nightingale Training School for Nurses at St Thomas Hospital and wrote NOTES FOR NURSING as a text for nursing and administering hospitals. This book has been translated into nine languages and is still in print.

While reading about Florence Nightingale, I was surprised to find she was the first woman to be elected a Fellow of the Royal Statistical Society for the work she did using statistical evidence to prove a point.   For example, she used a "polar-area diagram" or "coxcomb", as she called it, to demonstrate the causes of death of the soldiers in Scutari over a twelve month period. "In 1874, the American Statistical Association elected her an honorary member" (Kopf, Edwin W.   "Florence Nightingale as Statistician." Studies in the History of Statistics-Probability, New York Macmillan Publishing Co. Inc 1977) She had the ability to view a situation and determine solutions to problems. Her life spanned the years from 1820 to 1910 during the time when the foundations for modern hospitals were first developed.   She had ideas on how hospitals should be built allowing for windows, fresh air and reducing crowded conditions.   Her tools were the importance of cleanliness and providing resources to get the job done. She was interested in the big picture of providing a place where medical care could be safely carried out. This then was the first step towards modern medical and nursing care.

Note: The above information on the life of Florence Nightingale came from an article titled "Florence Nightingale" from the website for the Nightingale Museum in London, England.

FOREWORD

The body of this narrative begins in September of 1941, however, September 1, 1939 drastically changed our way of living so here I find I must digress again and give a not so brief explanation describing the times in which we lived, thus setting the stage, so to speak.

My family lived on a ranch in the brush country area of Southwest Texas twenty-five miles west of Uvalde. Eagle Pass, a small, isolated, and dusty town, was thirty five miles west of us on the banks of the Rio Grande River which separates the United States from Mexico. Uvalde is on Highway 90 which connects San Antonio to El Paso. We did most of our shopping and business in Uvalde in 1939. Our family group and employees created an almost self-sustaining unit. There were five dwelling houses on the ranch. The headquarters home was an airy two story wooden structure with a basement and a widow's walk on the peaked roof. In 1941 my four brothers, two of whom were married, a sister, our parents and myself completed the family circle on the ranch. Each week someone from the ranch went to Uvalde by car on the unpaved road to pick up the general delivery mail, buy groceries and other supplies for everyone. Our business was ranching with some irrigated farming to raise supplemental feed-stuff for the cattle. We built dirt tanks for other ranchers under a government program and hired men to drive the heavy dirt-moving equipment. My father, also, always had bees and raised honey and sold the surplus.

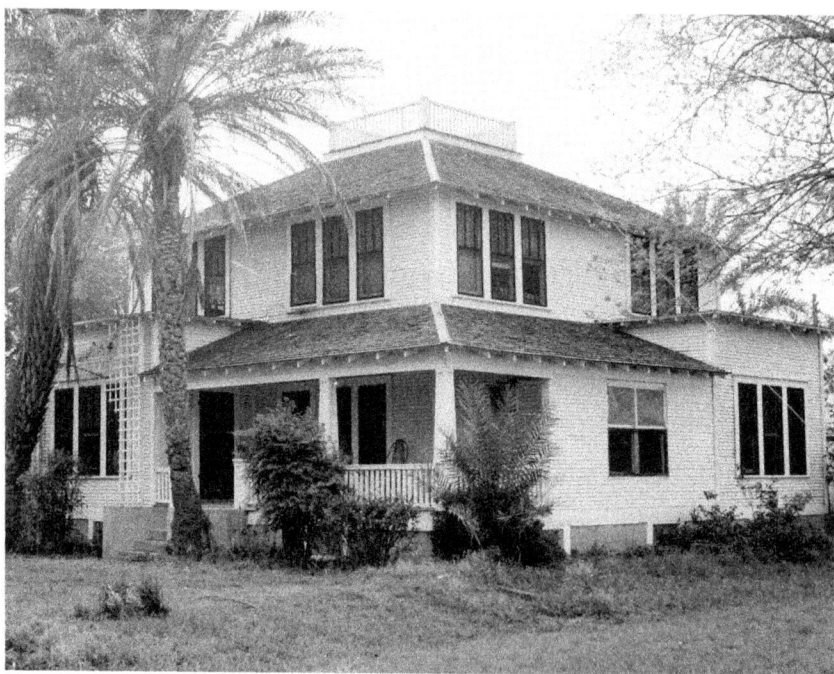

(The ranch house in later years. Photo Credit: Ernest Franke)

In the years prior to 1941 we lived in a pre-TV, pre-credit card, and pre-plastic, pre-landfill world. News arrived via newspapers and radio. Air-conditioning did not exist in either cars or homes. The Untied States was trying to recover from the Great Depression of the nineteen thirties (1930s). Wages were low and not everyone had a job. Fortunately, we lived in an agrarian society and in many cases grown children returned to their parents' farm and worked there until they found another job. Prior to 1939 my father hired married men with families on the ranch in Maverick County, Texas, for $1.00 a day plus housing, a garden plot and milk. My father could not afford to pay more and the men were willing to work for that wage while having a safe place to bring their families to live until times were better. As one president had said "Make do, use it up, do without." At that time people were adept at "making do" with what they had. Actually, they had little choice. Innovation became the practice of the day. For one example many a dress, shirt, curtain, bedspread or dish-towel was made from printed cotton sacks that had held chicken feed. Whoever bought the feed was commissioned to buy sacks of feed with matching prints.

I vividly remember the morning of September 1, 1939. My brother, Arthur, had been the County Surveyor for Maverick County. He headed our crew building dirt tanks under a government program. These dirt tanks provided watering holes for cattle and wildlife and replaced water wells which when dug in our semi-arid countryside were often "dry", meaning they did not produce water. Arthur decided to have a picnic and to invite all the ranchers for whom he and his crew had built tanks. He picked September 1, 1939 for the day. We had boiled potatoes the day before and early on the morning of September the first we were busily cutting up onions and potatoes for potato salad when we heard our sister-in-law running across our caliche croquet court from her house shouting, "Hitler has invaded Poland." She had one of the few radios on the ranch. What a shocking thing to hear and we, of course, wondered what would happen next. The barbecue picnic took place as planned on the banks of the Chaparosa Creek under large oak trees near the ranch headquarters. As the invitees arrived each received a "raspa" (flavored shaved ice) to cool themselves after their long dusty trip. I remember the men clustered around a car radio while they listened to the horrendous news. The news certainly dampened our spirits. The great unknown lay before us.

The following days were dramatic. On the third of September Prime Minister Chamberlain of Great Britain declared a state of war against Germany. By October the 6th of 1939, Poland no longer existed as a country. President Franklin D. Roosevelt, in his second term as president, signed the Selective Training and Service Act of 1940. The Act created the first peacetime draft and formally established the Selective Service System as an independent

Federal agency.   Registration for the draft took place on April 2, 1942, registering men born on or after April 1877 or before 16th of April 1897. All men from ages 18 to 45 and 45 to 65 were eligible to be registered. Only the 18 to 45 year old men were registered and drafted. This draft became known as the 4th draft. The first draft occurred during the Civil War in 1861--1865.

After registration for the draft and calling up of the young single men, only my married brothers and a married cousin remained as workers at the ranch. They were considered to be working in an essential industry.   The methods used in the ranching operation changed because of less help.   For example, since baling hay required at least eight people with the equipment available, that task was eliminated.   One cowboy working with several Border Collie dogs replaced a group of cowboys.

Permit me to digress here a moment. The CCC or Civilian Conservation Corps started in 1933 by President Franklin Roosevelt during the first 100 days of his first term gave employment to many young men at the depth of the depression. Each man sent $25.00 of their $30.00 check home which in turn gave a lift to the economy. (What effect, you ask, could $25.00 have on the economy! We forget or do not realize how the value of money has changed through the years.) The young men had an active outdoor life helping with reforestation and the building of facilities in state and national parks. All of this turned out to be excellent training for the military where most of these young men finally went. We had one young man working at the ranch who constantly told us "When I was in the CCC camp I did ...." until we were quite tired of his stories. When the war began my squirrel and coon hunting cousins became marksmen in the army. My cousins who had graduated from the Corps at A&M University at College Station, Texas became officers in the Infantry or as Paratroopers.

One of my unmarried brothers was drafted, and the other one volunteered. Arthur became a sergeant arriving in France on D 2 day and rode in a jeep carrying maps and billeted officers in Germany. He ended his stay in Europe at Aachen, Germany. Sidney became a truck driver on the blacked-out California coast and later drove trucks in France.

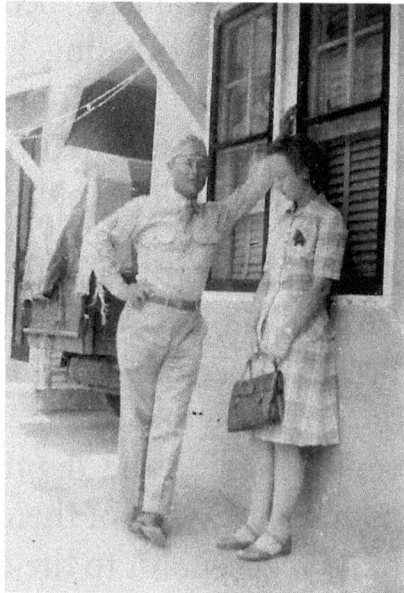

(Arthur and Bea in Abeline, Tx. after the war)

Wars throughout history have caused economies to prosper with the need for the production of more and newer products. As this tale unfolds we will read about many of these products. The struggling economy turned around when shipbuilding began and with the manufacturing of goods needed for the war effort. The men and their families from the ranch moved to the Houston, Texas area where they helped build ships and received increased wages. The homes and real estate they bought likewise escalated in prices during the following years. Tom Brokaw, a twenty year television anchorman with the National Broadcasting Company, wrote a book THE GREATEST GENERATION. He interviewed survivors of D day and praised them for their courage and their later achievements. Those of us who survived those times over the long haul benefited from those times as well. Under the GI Bill veterans received many benefits, if they made use of them, consisting of college tuition (including books and a living stipend), low interest loans for houses and low interest loans up to $10,000 for rural land purchases (at that time land was inexpensive compared to later).

When I think back to those days I realize how amazingly uninformed and unaware of the world situation I had been in September of 1941. Perhaps it is after the fact, when history tells us what happened, that we finally comprehend the ramifications of the times. At nineteen years of age I had finished two years of college at Texas Lutheran Junior College in Seguin, Texas, where I had taken courses in science and education and had been trying to decide between nursing and teaching which were the professions approved for women at that time along with secretarial work. Many of my friends who had taken typing and shorthand became Civil Service workers for the Federal Government. Although I could type and take shorthand I had discovered I did not care for that type of work. I felt inadequate to teach since teachers seemed always to be saying, "This is the way it is," and I wasn't always sure it was that way. I knew two plus two was four but what about all the unknowns? After my experience as Editor of THE LONE STAR LUTHERAN at Texas Lutheran Junior College in Seguin, I really wanted to become a writer but I had the feeling I should experience life before attempting to write about life. So off I went to Galveston to take the three-year course to become a Registered Nurse.

I ARRIVE IN GALVESTON, TEXAS

I arrived in Galveston, Texas in September of 1941 on a windy, blustery day amidst hurricane warnings. After a quick lunch at a restaurant on the seawall with waves breaking higher and higher, my brothers Arthur and Sidney and sister Gertrude deposited me at the residence of the John Sealy College of Nursing where I would spend the next three years. The University of Texas had a Medical School and a Nursing School at the John Sealy Hospital in Galveston, and I was entering the Nursing School. Earlier that morning the four of us had driven across the two-mile causeway bridge connecting the mainland with Galveston Island. The water was already rough and a threatening sky covered us. On arrival at the Nurses' Residence I quickly removed my belongings from the car and my brothers and sister left for Houston because the news on the radio already reported the causeway bridge might be closed at any moment, and then they would not be able to leave the island. My siblings spent the night in Houston with our father's brother Rudolph Franke and his wife Julia. As the hurricane hit, my sister wondered if she would ever see me again.

Many steps led up to the Rebecca Sealy Nurses Residence. I felt welcomed to my destination. I knew I had arrived! The sister of a student I had known in Uvalde High School met me on the steps. Agnes Cox said she had heard someone was coming from Uvalde and was watching for me. She was in her senior year and knew her way around and, therefore, was of great help to me. Agnes and I located my room and I moved in. Single rooms were provided for each student and were furnished with a single bed, dresser, desk with bookcase, clothes closet and washbasin with mirror above it. Bathrooms and showers were communal. A tall palm tree grew outside my room's second story window. During that night and the following years I

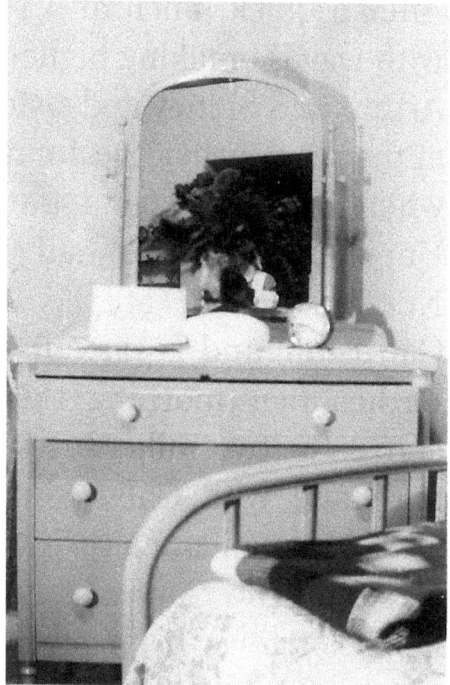

(Furnishings in Bea's dorm room with bouquet of red roses on the dresser)

watched the movement of the palm's fronds while the annual hurricanes roared. After my first morning and many other mornings I was glad to see the palm tree still stood upright.

When I arrived in 1941, the John Sealy Nurses' Residence, built in 1932 to accommodate 163 nurses, was a very pleasant, well-equipped building. The front doors of the residence opened into a large foyer with the mailboxes on the right next to the residence director's office. Directly in front of the entrance beyond the foyer was a large reception room with a piano, fireplace, radio, numerous comfortable chairs and sofas and a large table from which we occasionally were served afternoon tea. I remember the evening gatherings we used to have there while we listened to President Roosevelt's "fireside chats" on the radio during the World War II years. To the left of the foyer was an elevator which, according to custom, upper classmates always entered first.

From a day-room on the second floor we could enter a patio on the roof covering the first floor reception room. This outdoor patio made a great place to sunbathe or sit and relax in the mornings or late evenings. During the war years curfews and black-outs were often in place. When an order for a black-out was issued black shades on each window were pulled down so no interior lights could be seen from outside the buildings. After the Japanese bombing of Pearl Harbor in Hawaii on December 7, 1941 and our entry into the war with Germany and Japan, there was great concern for the safety of everyone. Rumors of German U boats (submarines) in the Gulf of Mexico increased these concerns. Often bananas and other debris would be found on the beach and we would speculate what kind of boat or ship had been sunk.

The auditorium, reception room, nursing school offices and classrooms occupied most of the first floor of the residence. In the Nursing Arts Lab the pre-clinical students learned all the basic patient care procedures including how to give intra-muscular injections with a glass hypodermic syringe and small gauge needle—first into an orange and then into each other's arms. Our Procedure Book included throat irrigations and other procedures which were soon no longer needed with the advent of Penicillin.

THE MAKING OF AN RN

If I remember correctly, tuition of $312.00 covered all my expenses for the three years I was in Galveston. At the time, the staffing in the John Sealy Hospital consisted of registered nurses (RNs) as Head Nurses for the units from 7 a.m. to 3 p.m. hours with a few evening registered nurses from 3 p.m. to 11 p.m. RNs staffed the Operating Rooms. The more experienced student nurses provided the majority of the staffing from 3 p.m. to 11 p.m. and 11 p.m. to 7 a.m. under the supervision of an evening and night supervisor. We were trained to be responsible for our units and received excellent clinical experience for the times. In 1941, John Sealy had the reputation of providing one of the best learning experiences available for student nurses in the state of Texas.

The John Sealy Training School for Nurses opened on March 10, 1890. Fifty-one years later I entered the school. The students rotated through all the areas of the hospital: medical, surgical, pediatrics, obstetrics and gynecology, operating room, psychiatry, emergency room, outpatient clinics, and diet kitchen. Our pictures were included in THE

CACTUS, the annual of the University of Texas in Austin. In the 1942 CACTUS, my pre-clinical class picture included 69 students. We did not receive college credit from the University of Texas. A number of my classmates had been teachers with Bachelor's Degrees before they entered nurses training. All of us had to take Chemistry as it applied to nursing even though we had taken Chemistry in college. The emphasis was different.

However, when I matriculated in 1947 at Incarnate Word College in San Antonio I received twenty-four credits for my three years in Galveston or approximately one-fourth of the credits I needed for a Bachelor of Science in Nursing Education. Incarnate Word accepted all my credits from Texas Lutheran College. After an additional attendance of twelve months at Incarnate Word College I received my degree. At the time of admission to Incarnate Word, I was a registered nurse with about four years experience in nursing including fourteen months in the Army Nurse Corps (from 1945-1946, which is another story).

Each student had a rotation schedule that moved her through the various specialties. Our level of education determined when we would proceed. The medical-surgical areas were the first to be offered, and others followed. Occasionally, a need for personnel caused a student to enter a specialty before she had received the class instruction. This happened to me when I had my psychiatric experience. (More about that later.)

As we gained clinical experience the appearance of our uniforms changed. During our pre-clinical period our uniform consisted of a blue chambray dress with a separate white apron both to mid-calf with white cuffs which we pinned to the short blue sleeves of the dress. The white collar buttoned to the blue neckline in the center back and then brought to the front of the neckline and fastened inside with safety pins. The chambray dress had pearl-like buttons with shanks secured on the underside after the button was punched through an eyelet in the dress. The uniform included white cotton stockings and white shoes. During the war years the United States government annually gave each citizen a ration book which included coupons for sugar, gasoline, and three pairs of shoes. Shoes to wear with our nursing uniforms were of primary concern, and we often needed most of the shoe allotment for uniform shoes. Huaraches, a type of leather woven shoe made in Mexico, not on the ration list, became our shoe for casual use.

During the first six months, designated the pre-clinical period, the students were taught the basic patient care procedures and then were given an opportunity to practice the procedures on a medical unit. Also, we had been taught some of the back-ground of professional nursing including an introduction to Florence Nightingale and Clara Barton. We felt we were becoming a part of the story of improved nursing care.

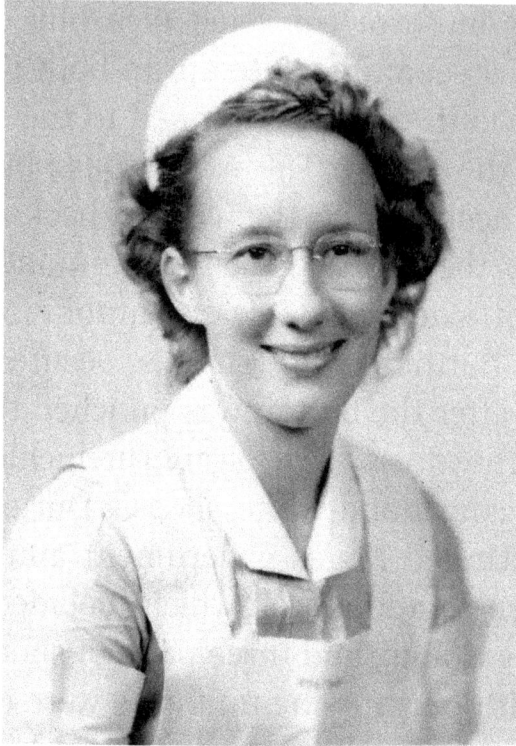

(Bea in her student dress, apron, and cap)

At the end of the pre-clinical period each of the students received her cap during a "capping ceremony." This was a very solemn ceremony. The caps placed on a table in a long orderly line awaited us. A lighted replica of a lamp similar to one used in Florence Nightingale's time sat on the table from which each student lit her individual candle after receiving her cap. Then as a group we recited the Florence Nightingale pledge which follows:

"I solemnly pledge myself before God and in the presence of the assembly, to pass my life in purity and to practice my profession faithfully. I will abstain from whatever is deleterious and mischievous and will not take or knowingly administer any harmful drug. I will do all in my power to maintain and elevate the standard of my profession, and will hold in confidence all personal matters committed to my keeping and all family affairs coming to my knowledge in the practice of my calling. With loyalty will I endeavor to aid the physician, in his work, and devote myself to the welfare of those committed to my care."

Note: "The Nightingale Pledge was composed by Lystra Gretter, an instructor of nursing at the old Harper Hospital in Detroit, Michigan, and was first used by its graduating class in the spring of 1893. It is an adaptation of the Hippocratic Oath taken by physicians." (I found this notation on the internet which quoted from A SHORT HISTORY OF NURSING by Lavinia Dock and Isabel Stuart.)

The capping ceremony marked the culmination of an arduous training period. Needless to say those of us who had survived the pre-clinical period were very happy to receive our caps and looked forward to the rest of our education to become registered nurses. The next day when we reported to work all decked out in the full uniform of clinical student nurses, our patients welcomed us by clapping their hands. Then patients remained in the hospital for enough time for us to develop a friendly relation with each other.

The day of the capping ceremony, prior to the program, each student received the bib for her apron so she could wear it that evening. The waistline of the apron consisted of the usual waist-band with a second inner band to which we pinned the bib. The straps of the bib went over the shoulders and after being crossed were then pinned to the waist band with the apron buttoning in the middle of the back. Setting up a uniform with all the buttons and pinning required quite a bit of time. The bib had a tape on the center front with each student nurse's name on it. I remember standing in my room in front of my dresser arranging my uniform and looking into the mirror, and there I saw my reflection and on my bib a mirror image of my name, Miss Franke, which reflected backward "eknarF ssiM" with each letter reversed as well. I must say the past six months had been different and seeing my name spelled backward in the mirror capped (no pun intended) it all. My family had sent a bouquet of red roses for this big event in my life and I stood there for a moment admiring the reflection of the roses and Miss Franke spelled backwards. *(Editor: Notice the bouquet of roses on the dresser in the picture on page 2.)* The John Sealy cap had a rounded bill attached to a piece of material which had a drawstring which when pulled shaped the cap with the bill turned up and tilted back. We could then secure the cap to our hair on top of our head. The original $312.00 tuition included laundry service. Each week the soiled uniforms were bundled into a laundry bag and later the uniforms were returned all beautifully washed and starched. I can still hear the call in the hallway by students "The uniforms are here, the uniforms are here," and we would rush to pick ours up and start pinning them together.

In those days, and for many years afterward, the cap symbolized Professional Nursing care and personal dedication to the art and science of nursing following the Nightingale precepts. Caps varied according to each nursing school. One of our instructors, Miss White, graduated from Philadelphia General Hospital. We all gasped the first time we saw her in uniform. Her cap, which was quite small with crimped fluting around the edge, was perched on top of her head. The instructor noticed our interest, removed it from her head and talked about the cap. I thought she handled the situation quite well.

As I remember the rules for wearing a cap were given as: no nurse should ever wear the cap while driving a car and never should a nurse smoke a cigarette with a cap on her head. The cap was to be put in place on one's head when the nurse entered the unit where she worked. Usually in the Catholic schools of nursing the senior students received a black band to be attached to their cap. Later, when I was Director of Nursing Service at Santa Rosa Hospital in San Antonio, occasionally I would find a Sealy nurse with a black band on her cap. When I asked her about the black band she said when working in a Catholic hospital without a black band many people thought she was an undergraduate so she had added the band to clarify her standing!

A graduation ceremony marked the end of the academic work; however, each student had to complete her three years to the day in nursing school. Some students did not take vacation and completed in August. The rest of us who had taken vacation time or had been ill completed our allotted time at John Sealy at a later date. I finished in 1944 on September 21st. A custom, which some people might consider strange, had been handed down through the years. During the three years each student received new uniforms as needed but by the time she had "put in her time" most of the blue chambray dress part of the uniform was washed out, thin and faded. The last morning the student reported for duty in her oldest uniform and worked until about eleven o'clock. On her way to the residence to put on her new white graduate uniform her fellow student nurses tore her old student uniform from her body leaving enough of it in place so she was decently clad.

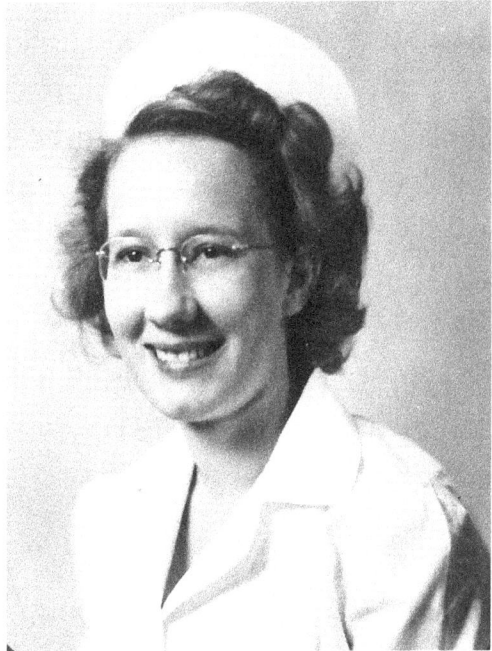

(Bea in her new nursing uniform and cap after graduation)

At noon, dressed in her new white uniform with cap, she reported to the cafeteria where a table awaited the new graduate honoree, her guests, and the Dean of the School of Nursing.

Sometime during the last few months of our senior experience the senior class as a group went to Houston to take the State Board Examination. Several months after graduation each of us received notification whether we passed or failed the State Boards. You can imagine the joy I felt when I received notification I had passed. I really did not think failure was possible; however, receiving the passing notice finalized the three years. With the registration of my certificate at the Bexar County Courthouse in San Antonio, Texas, I became a Registered Nurse (RN). During the interim between graduation and registration I worked as a graduate nurse with the understanding I was awaiting State Board notification. My first job was in the operating room of the Nix Hospital in San Antonio, as a circulating and scrub nurse as we were designated then. I received one hundred and fifty dollars ($150.00) a month which was considered a good salary at that time. (This is another example of the changing value of money if compared with 2011 salaries.)

LEARNING THE ART OF NURSING

One of the first classes given to the pre-clinical students included a brief history of Galveston. The city of Galveston is on an island which gives it a uniqueness. The American Automobile Association's Tour Book of 1995 recounts a brief history of Galveston. "In 1817 Jean Lafitte and his pirates took over the abandoned base of a Mexican revolutionary and renamed it Campeachy..... Campeachy was abandoned and burned when the United States forced Lafitte to leave in 1821..... Renamed Galveston for Bernardo de Galvez, a Spanish Governor of the Louisiana Territory and an ally of the United States during the American Revolution. The former pirate stronghold became the Republic's base of naval operations against Mexico and the temporary Texas capital in 1836. By the Civil War, Galveston was Texas' principal seaport and leading commercial center, and by 1890 it was Texas' largest and wealthiest city....Galveston lost everything to the hurricane of 1900, in which some 6,000 persons died.....Despite a massive engineering feat that in some places raised the city 17 feet behind a 10 mile long seawall, Galveston lost its former status to its expanding neighbor, Houston." I remember a building known as LaFitte's house within walking distance of the hospital.

The city of Galveston was laid out with the streets named with alphabets running the length of the island and streets with numbers crossing them, thus making the location of places in the city very easy. Grace Decker, one of our instructors, taught a course dubbed Sociology in which she described our immediate area. She told us how to conduct ourselves since some areas were considered safer than others. I remember particularly we were told Post-Office Street or F included a "red light" district and in other areas of town there were some gambling "dens." Post-Office Street paralleled Mechanic or D, the street on which the Rebecca Sealy Nurses Residence was built. We were advised when we went to town to go with a friend or in a group. The beach, only about eight blocks from the residence, at Seawall and Broadway, was easily accessible. During the first two and one-half years we

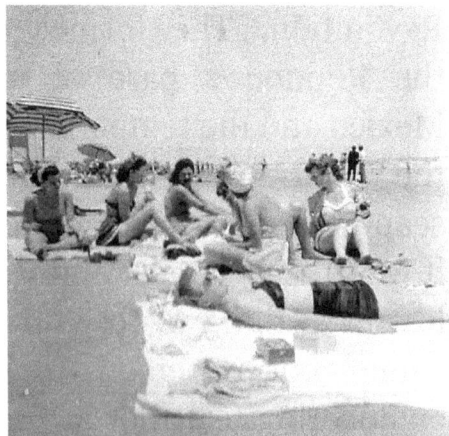

(Nursing School classmates relaxing on the beach)

could only go to the beach during the day since blackouts during the war kept it closed at night. The last half-year my friends and I went to the beach at night since the U boat dangers no longer existed, and there was no longer a curfew. I remember swimming out on the moon-lit path at night. Galveston was an old beautiful city with colorful oleanders, hibiscus and palm trees. Broadway, the main street running the length of the island from the causeway to the Seawall at Stewart Beach, was a boulevard with palm trees interspersed with oleanders and hibiscus in the middle. We enjoyed walking down this shaded area.

The pre-clinical nursing students learned the basic nursing procedures in the Nursing Arts Laboratory equipped with all the equipment needed for patient care. Notice the term Nursing Arts! The instructors constantly drilled into us that our foremost concern must be the care and well being of the patient. The practice of patient care, then, was considered an art. Each student received a Procedure Book in which she placed her learned procedures. I found my book from 1941 to 1944 recently and leafed through it. This tome is a period piece! The book describes personal patient care and also, directions for using the equipment of the time. The patient care procedures are still relevant. However, after more than sixty years much of the equipment is, of course, out-dated and has not been used for years, having been replaced by newer medicines and technologies. However, in 1941 this was the way patient care and medicine was practiced. We were at the cutting edge in our time as, I think, all times are on the cutting edge. A perceived need makes a procedure necessary. Materials available will determine the type of equipment to be used, and the science of medicine and the art of nursing will determine what procedure will be done. The cutting edge is always "now," and change occurs when someone is able to recognize a need and determines a method suitable for the times using the materials and knowledge available to perform the new or revised task in a more efficient way.

Our education began with cleaning beds after a patient went home. We were taught how to make closed, open, fracture, occupied, ether, emergency, and cradle beds. At that time there were few people in the housekeeping staff, so we were taught housekeeping duties as well. (Perhaps, I should point out the time of which I write was before nurse aides, orderlies, and Licensed Vocational Nurses worked in hospitals.)

Next we learned how to give bed baths and evening and morning care. The evening care consisted of "care of mouth and teeth, offer bed pan, wash hands and face, give care to the back, change linen if necessary, brush crumbs out of bed with bath towel or whisk broom, if lower sheet is not changed, loosen at side and tighten, shake and replace pillows, straighten top covers, wash pitcher and fill with ice water and leave patient comfortable." Early ambulation may have done away with backrubs but the comfort of one once experienced is long remembered.

In those days we were taught to give the patients good basic nursing care. One procedure named "For The Comfort Of The Patient" includes the aim "To make and keep the patient comfortable." (What patient would not desire and deserve comfort!) Following are the

GENERAL INSTRUCTIONS:

1. Work evenly and smoothly. Use long even strokes.
2. The touch should be firm, gentle and effective.
3. Use the whole hand, not fingers only. Hands should be smooth, warm and dry.
4. Avoid jerking or jarring a patient.
5. Never discuss a patient's condition in her presence, even though the patient may be unconscious.
6. Never discuss a patient's condition with another patient.

7. Satisfy the questions of patients, whenever possible, in accordance with good judgment and common sense.

8. Never go out of a room without leaving it in better condition and more agreeable to the patient and with a happier atmosphere than when you entered.

9. When possible, complete a piece of work leaving it in a finished condition, before starting another piece of work.

10. Sources of discomfort
    a) Bad ventilation.
    b) Noise, loud voices, whispering, hard heels, squeaky shoes, leaking faucets, banging doors, squeaking hinges.
    c) If the patient is in one position too long.
    d) Extremes of temperature.
    e) Lack of cleanliness.
    f) Weight and pressure on sensitive parts— wrinkled bedding.

The first three statements under General Instructions listed above refer to the placement of the nurse's hands on the patient maintaining a constant and firm touch while giving a back rub or bed bath. (Here I should add we did not wear rubber gloves when giving bedside care in those days. We actually touched the patient. Also, I remember how the patients enjoyed having their draw sheet, a half sheet under their buttocks, pulled tightly and any crumbs removed from their bed. These were small points but were helpful for the patient's comfort when hospitalized for a long time. Making comparisons between times is tempting, but I shall try to refrain from doing so.)

It might be well to point out we had many orthopedic patients who then required   lengthy stays. Many patients had Thompson splints on a leg with a pin through the knee area. These were city or county patients being treated by the surgical staff. Patients who had their hernias repaired remained in bed for a week or more. Obstetrical patients stayed in the hospital for a few days and remained in bed at home for another week.

Included in our book were nursing procedures such as various types of bandaging; irrigations such as colonic, ear, eye, nasal, throat, vaginal; application of heat including fomentations, turpentine stupes, flaxseed poultices, mustard plaster, foot baths, mustard foot bath, local hot air bake, hot pack; application of cold such as ice pack, cool sponge bath, and cold packs.

A four-page procedure described the isolation technique used to protect other patients. Frequently, pneumonia patients or patients with suppurating deep burns were isolated in the wards with the use of portable screens, and gowns, and basins of solutions for the nurse or doctor to wash their hands. The Main Building, built in 1890 and rebuilt after the 1900 storm, had limited plumbing facilities and limited electrical outlets. Facilities available always affect how procedures can be done. We did the best we could with the existing limitations and always were told, "If you don't have what you need improvise." Enclosed porches provided space to isolate tubercular patients (TB). Typhoid patients, if possible, were placed in private rooms, and in each case the basic isolation technique used was modified according to the accommodations available.

Here is an example of how nursing has changed. In 1941-1944, we shaved the surgical area on patients the day prior to the day of surgery. The description of this procedure appears in the book as "Preparation of the Field of Surgery" and dated 5/2/40. The purpose includes

1. To stimulate the skin glands in order to promote a profuse secretion which will wash bacteria out of ducts.

2. To dissolve the sebaceous secretion of the skin surface by the use of a fat solvent (ether, benzine or alcohol).

3. To remove dissolved fat, disintegrated epithelial cells, and bacteria.

4. To check secretions by the use of ether.

While I was in the Army Nurse Corps during 1945 and 1946, patients were shaved the evening before surgery with sterile towels placed over the shaved area. Later, when I worked at the Nix Hospital in San Antonio, we did the shaving prior to surgery in the operating room. I became remarkably adept with a straight razor.

The beliefs concerning the germ theory seemed to change continually and, probably still continue to do so. I found a quote from THE HISTORY OF THE TEXAS MEDICAL ASSOCIATION 1853–1953 written by Dr. P.I. Nixon. On page 199 the author quotes a Dr. Thomas Pugh: "The success of the operation (tonsillectomy performed on the back porch) without regard to the aseptic regime certainly knocks out that fad." This statement got my attention since my father had told my mother their family doctor had lined up his brothers and sisters and removed their tonsils on the front porch of their house in the country. He was born in 1873. My mother never believed this tale.

In Galveston each unit had a Doctor's Order Book in which each doctor wrote his orders and from it the orders were transcribed to the patient's chart and then to the Kardex and to medicine and treatment cards. (I remember in the early 1950s employing a mature, intelligent woman to be trained as our first ward clerk at Santa Rosa Hospital in San Antonio. She was assigned to the post-partum unit since many of the doctors with patients on that unit used standing orders and the work would be less complicated for her on that unit than on some of the other units. Hiring this first ward clerk was a learning experience for both the staff and for her and turned out completely successful saving a great deal of time for the nurses.)

The patient's chart included a graph sheet for temperatures, pulse, and respiration graphed in blue ink; blood pressures in red ink; and weight and height in the designated area in red ink; intake and output totals written on graph sheet by night nurse at 6 a.m.; stool recorded at 8 a.m. in black ink. At midnight the night nurse would draw a red line closing the previous 24 hours. This graph sheet gave a quick over-view of the vital signs of a patient.

Our curriculum included a short class in printing by hand as all notations on the nurses' notes were to be printed. We learned to print quite quickly. (No computers then.)

Also included in the procedure book were the set-ups for the equipment; then we stood by while a doctor, resident, intern, or medical student completed the procedure.

For example hypodermaclysis or clysis is included in the procedure book. A "clysis" was a slow drip injection of large amounts of normal saline (.9 %) introduced through a 19 gauge by 3 inch long needle into the thigh muscles or with shorter needles into the back of the patient. This procedure was frequently used for children. Doctors always started a clysis. Intra-venous fluids were beginning to replace the clysis, and I can imagine the patients were happy with that change.

The infusion procedure states, "An intravenous infusion consists of the introduction of an isotonic solution into the vein." If a solution was to be added to the isotonic solution a procedure describes how this was to be done. At that time intravenous solutions were made in the operating room. The glass bottles were reused, solutions mixed, and solution and bottle autoclaved with a temporary gauze stopper which was replaced with a sterile screw top when cool.

The rubber tubing for IVs was reused after being carefully washed, dried and wrapped in a muslin wrapper and then autoclaved (dry heat for a designated length of time). Medical students started the IVs to obtain practice. We were familiar with the procedure but were not given the opportunity to practice it as the medical students needed the practice. There is a reference in my procedure book to Cutter solution which is the name of probably the first company to prepare solutions for intravenous use commercially. Before companies participate in producing supplies and equipment there must be a demonstrated need and an opportunity for profit.

It is interesting to note at that time needles were re-sharpened with a whetstone when they became dull and boiled on the unit in a small sterilizer before use. The gauge of the needles were larger then, which made entering veins more difficult.

Rubber gloves were washed, turned inside out, washed again, dried, turned, dried, powdered with talcum powder inside and out and placed in a glove wrapper with two pockets. A right hand glove was placed in the pocket on the right and a left hand glove placed in the left side pocket. These gloves in their pockets were then wrapped again in another muslin wrapper and autoclaved. At that time gloves and tubing was all made of rubber and recycled. The gloves were labeled according to size before being autoclaved. Disposable plastic tubing did not appear in hospitals until the 1950s as I remember.

There are many types of irrigations described in this 60+ year old procedure book including throat irrigations, soon displaced by medications. Some types of irrigations were continued for many years. One of these procedures which worked by the laws of physics describes the set up and use of a "tidal irrigation" following prostate surgery. The procedure includes the drawing of two bottles with a "y" shaped glass connector attached to rubber tubing with two ends of the tubing connected to two bottles, one on a standard filled with a solution and the other below the level of the patient and the third end connected to the catheter to the patient. The opening and closing of two clamps, one on each piece of tubing connecting the bottles to the catheter, controlled the flow of the solution. With this setup the bladder could be irrigated with a specific amount of fluid at stated times to keep clots from forming. Again, years later, with improvement in surgical technique this procedure became decreasingly used and abandoned. For a time irrigations with asepto syringes were done.

Another procedure named "Continuous Upper Intestinal Decompression" describes the setup and use of the Wangensteen suction. This suction device is "named after Dr. Wangensteen at the University of Minnesota who with his associates developed an apparatus for the continuous suction and aspiration of the stomach contents." To further quote: "This simple procedure has practically revolutionized intestinal surgery, allowing extensive work to be done without danger of it breaking down and without the fear of death from the formerly dreaded ileus. The gases in the bowel, other than a very minimum amount formed in the natural putrefactive process, is swallowed air. Death from ileus is invariably due to the loss of the function from interference in the circulation of the bowel from distention." The John Sealy apparatus was a modification of the original idea and "the principle that an ordinary siphon with a reservoir of water to maintain the flow and also act as a chamber for the collection of the aspirated gaseous contents." A detailed picture of the apparatus is included in the procedure book. When sulfa drugs became available they were given for several days prior to intestinal surgery. Our Procedure Book, also, included paracentesis, thoracentesis and other procedures.

During the Pre-Clinical period we were also introduced to massage through a ten hour course. According to Tappan's HEALING MASSAGE TECHNIQUES by Frances M. Tappan and Patricia J. Benjamin published by Appleton & Lange Stamford, CT page 77, "Western massage techniques are methods of soft tissue manipulation developed in Europe and the United States over the past two centuries." The five technique categories are: effleurage, petrissage, friction, tapotement, and vibration. I had forgotten about effleurage which is a sliding or gliding movement which we probably used predominately in backrubs. Actually the only massage we probably did was backrubs. Physiotherapy was in its infancy at that time. The nurses helped patients learn to use crutches and canes. I don't remember if there were any walkers used for support for patients. (Sometimes when I write down my remembrances I feel I am reporting on the Dark Ages of Medicine, and I suppose those practicing in the field today would agree. I will state in our defense, older methods and techniques had predated 1941 to 1944 though it may seem impossible to the reader of the early 2000s. Methods and techniques constantly change and hopefully for the betterment of the patient.)

During the three years in Galveston we studied Principles and Practices of Nursing, Medical and Surgical Nursing, Pharmacology, Anatomy & Physiology, Chemistry, Pediatrics, Obstetrics and Gynecology, Psychiatry, Sociology, Dietetics, History of Nursing. One of our last courses was Professional Adjustments to prepare us for the place we would occupy as Registered Nurses.

The Professional Nurses Program included much helpful material but did not prepare us completely for what was to come. A year or so before we graduated the Federal Government established the Cadet Nurses Program. The students who joined the program received uniforms and a stipend and were expected to join the Army or Navy upon graduation. A number of my friends joined the program and did volunteer upon graduation. I did not take advantage of the program since I did not plan to join the military; however, six months after graduation I joined the Army Nurse Corps.

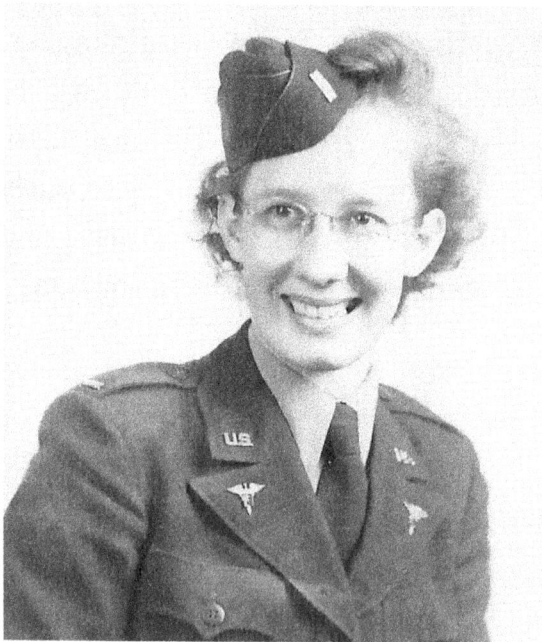

(Bea's Army Nurse uniform)

Permit me to digress here for a moment. After graduation I went to work at the Nix Hospital in San

Antonio, Texas in their Operating Room. There were a number of recent graduates working there. The administrator for the hospital was Miss Ellen Louise Brient. In January and February of 1945 the radio was constantly blaring about the need for nurses in the Army (this was before TV). Miss Brient kept telling all of the recent graduates we should join the army. I asked her how would the hospital manage without us and she assured me they would manage some way. At least four of us signed up and joined the large influx of new volunteers. Our numbers helped the military release nurses who had been in the hospital units on the front lines from North Africa through Italy and into France.

Later I met some of these nurses at Auburn General Hospital at McKinney, Texas. I remember one nurse at McKinney was afraid to walk from one building to another in the dark. They had put in their time and had done it well. I fought the "Battle of Texas", as I called it, for fourteen months and then was honorably discharged. We had completed caring for the returning veterans, and the great need for large numbers of nurses in the military was over. (My military experience is, also, another story— there are many stories!)

CLINICAL NURSING

Our instructors in Galveston told us how fortunate we were, for our work-day consisted of an eight hour day. Previously students and RNs worked a twelve hour day. Also, nurses worked six days a week then. (We started the five day week at Santa Rosa Hospital in San Antonio in the early 1950s which quite by accident coincided with the opening of the recovery room in that hospital.) As student nurses we worked either a straight 7 a.m. to 3 p.m. shift or a split shift (8 a.m. to 12 noon and 4 p.m. to 8. p.m.). This provided enough help on the units for serving the patients meals and giving morning and evening patient care. Whenever we had classes scheduled we went to them during the day even if we were working 3 p.m. to 11 p.m. or at night from 11 p.m. to 7 a.m. We found it most difficult to attend classes after working all night. Classes might be scattered throughout the day and you caught what sleep you could between classes and slept in the evening before reporting for duty at 11 p.m. When we had a split shift we were off from 12 noon to 4 p.m. We frequently walked about eight blocks to Stewart Beach for a few hours of relaxation in the sun and water before going back on duty at 4:00 p.m. Student nurses and one supervisor staffed the hospital at night. RNs were called in for emergency operations at night. Each unit had a 7:00 a.m. to 3:00 p.m. head nurse who worked a six-day week. By the time we completed this rigorous schedule, including clinical experience and classes for three years, we were well prepared to be in charge of a unit and do all the procedures required for that day and time.

When I recall my clinical experience I visualize no longer existing buildings peopled by many persons now long gone. This is a ghostlike experience in a way but at the time very real. As I move from building to building in my thoughts I remember many experiences which occurred in each of the buildings.

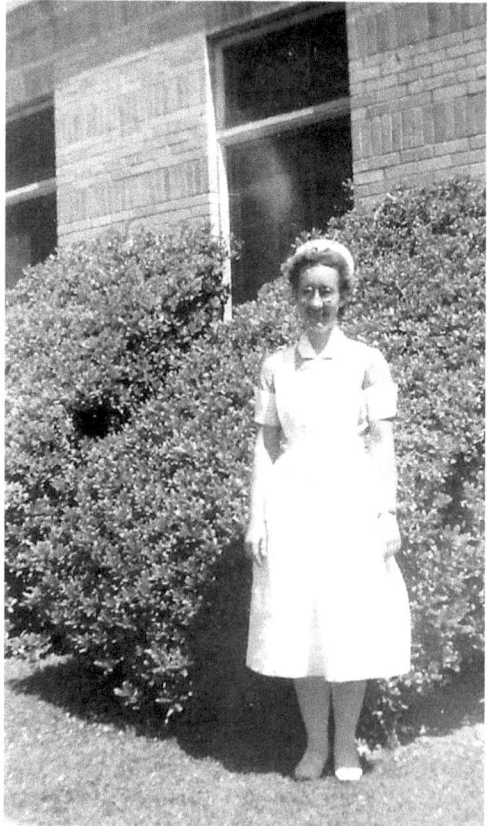

(Bea in full nurse's uniform outside one of the buildings)

Allow me to interject a bit of history here and quote from the book THE UNIVERSITY OF TEXAS BRANCH AT GALVESTON — A SEVENTY-FIVE YEAR HISTORY BY THE FACULTY AND STAFF published by the University of Texas Press, copyright 1967. "John Sealy, who died in 1884, provided for $50,000 to be devoted to a charitable purpose selected at the discretion of his brother, George Sealy, and his widow Rebecca Sealy. They chose to build the first John Sealy Hospital at a cost of $69,126.36." (page 15) The hospital provided facilities for over one hundred patients with wards and eight private rooms. The 1900 storm damaged it severely, and it had to be partially rebuilt. Throughout the following years the Sealy family, through the Sealy Smith Foundation, helped in many other financial ways including the building of the Rebecca Sealy Nurses Residence.

When I arrived the buildings of the John Sealy Hospital consisted of the Main Building, Women's Building, Children's Hospital, Clinic Building, Negro Hospital, Psychiatric Hospital, Isolation Building and of course, the Old Red Building.

"The construction of the Red Brick Building, which housed all the departments of the medical school, was begun in 1890" according to the above mentioned book A SEVENTY FIVE YEAR HISTORY of the University of Texas Medical Branch in

Galveston (page 21). Our pre-clinical class was taken to this building on one of our first tours of the hospital, and we walked through the dissection laboratory complete with cadavers and phenol odor as part of our tour. I often wondered if they were seeking out our "weaker sisters." Old Red, today, is the only building still standing and in use of all the buildings that were there when I was in Galveston.

The John Sealy Hospital opened on January 10, 1890. The Main Building was part of the original hospital. It consisted of a basement partially below ground with three floors above it. Offices filled part of the first floor, the cafeteria and a thirty bed men's ward. I am unsure what units were on the second floor. I believe there was a mixed medical-surgical unit for men on the third floor.

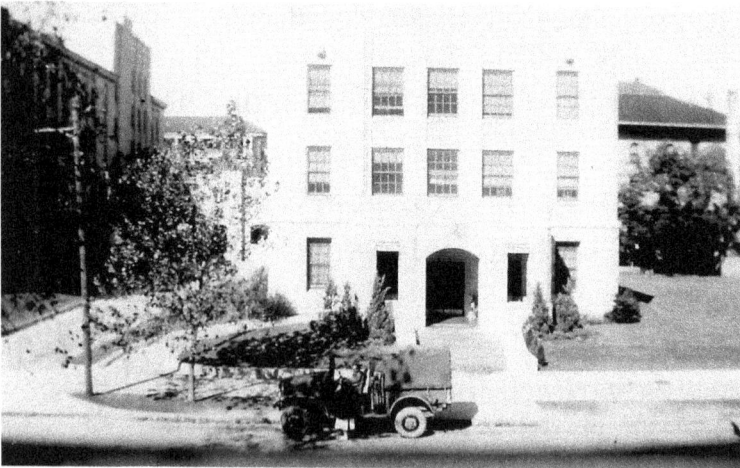

Several times during my three years I rotated to One Main, a thirty bed ward for men. The unit consisted of an enclosed porch with ten beds and another twenty beds inside. A bedside table separated each patient area. If a procedure required privacy, portable screens were pulled into place around the bed. At that time tuberculosis was a frequent disease and many times diagnosed after admission. In later years, for a time, every patient had a routine chest x-ray done on admission. Ten percent of the medical students and nursing students developed tuberculosis and required hospitalization or sanitarium care. Several of my classmates returned after being "cured" and completed their class and clinical work after we had finished. My skin test changed from a negative to a very strong positive affecting my entire upper arm, but my chest x-rays have always remained clear.

During one of my scheduled experiences on One Main, we had two gentlemen as patients who had cancer of the jaw and had been given massive jaw resection surgery. Each morning we would change their head dressings which consisted of placing a large pad against their exposed tongue held in place with roller bandages wrapped around and around their head and chin.

They received their nourishment by using an asepto syringe tipped with a short piece of rubber tubing which they inserted into their mouths and allowed the fluid to flow into their throats. This was before

Ensure; the mixture of tomato juice, milk, etc. was prepared in the Diet Kitchen. They were such patient fellows with such pleasant manners and seemed to take comfort in each other's companionship.

Let me now describe some of the equipment of our time. Our thermometer container consisted of a rack holding twenty test tubes each containing alcohol and one oral thermometer. After use, the thermometers were washed in soapy water (not hot as some of us found out!), rinsed and replaced in the alcohol where they were left for the appropriate time until the thermometers were re-sterilized. The alcohol was frequently replaced with fresh alcohol. Blood pressure sphygmomanometers were in portable cases.

In fact all equipment was portable. Oxygen tanks came from a central area and were wrestled into position. Oxygen tents consisting of a frame covered by a tent made out of treated cloth to retain the oxygen, with small windows made of a clear plastic-like material (isinglass?) so the nurse could observe the patient and the patient could see the nurse. The material of the tent was tucked under the head of the mattress and under the sides with the part over the abdomen folded with the top linens on the bed. Sometimes the doctor ordered nasal oxygen which was delivered through a single small gauge short rubber nasal tube placed in one nostril. To keep the tube in place the tube was bent upwards beside the exterior of the nose and fastened with adhesive tape to the forehead of the patient. This frequently was not a very secure method and if inserted incorrectly the patient's stomach might fill with air. When I think back, the type of materials available to make the equipment limited the equipment we used, and with new materials available new equipment can be made, and new procedures can be done. Plastic arrived at a later time and with it the two pronged plastic nasal oxygen tube in use later.

We were taught to defer to the doctors. As soon as a doctor arrived on the unit you acknowledged his presence and gave your chair to him if he required it. The doctor's orders were transferred from the Doctor's Order Book to a Kardex which consisted of a long vertical holder containing a collection of 3x5 cards with two for each patient, a day and night card, with the patient's current treatments and medications carefully recorded. At the changing of shifts this Kardex helped direct discussions concerning each patient. Medicine orders were transferred to cards which were then used when medications were poured. The medication nurse poured the medications into small glass medicine cups and then delivered the medication to each patient. These medicine glasses were washed and then boiled before being used again. (Years later at Santa Rosa we used disposable paper cups. We weren't into disposable in 1941–1944.) We used stock supplies of medication for the state and county patients. The private patients had their own supplies stored in the medication cabinet.

Each unit stored their narcotics in a locked cabinet. The nurse administering a narcotic signed out in the record book for the pill with time, name of patient and doctor ordering the pill. She would check the number of pills remaining against the number of pills used. At the end of each shift, after counting the supply, the nurse leaving and the one coming on cosigned the records. The nurse in charge was the keeper of the narcotic key. At that time morphine, codeine and dilaudid were in pill form and had to be converted to liquid form at the time of administration by placing the pill in a spoon-like device attached above an alcohol burner. The nurse added a few cubic centimeters of water to the spoon, dissolved the narcotic and, after cooling for a little while, the solution was pulled up into a glass syringe, the needle attached, and the injection given to the patient.

I will never forget the day when I arrived on One Main to give my first bed bath. The bedsteads were made of iron, tall at the head and short at the foot, with a small bedside table next to it. In the bedside table was a wash-basin, emesis-basin, soap dish, bar of soap, bedpan and urinal. The head nurse, I believe a Miss Sanders, introduced me to my patient who was in bed. I gathered my equipment together and placed it on a large tray—a basin of warm water, a bottle of alcohol for the backrub after the bath, a metal canister with powder to use after the backrub, and a bottle of liquor alkalinicus antisepticus used as a mouth wash after the patient brushed his teeth. I was dressed in my pre-clinical uniform and felt very new. I approached the patient carrying the tray of equipment. The water sloshed from side to side and the bottles rattled back and forth. I had been brought up if I was to do something I was to do it well. The patient, a pleasant fellow, had a very hairy chest. I applied soap and I scrubbed as we talked. At the time I didn't think about any soap I put on had to be removed, and that became a problem as the soap turned to lather. After many trips to the water faucet in the utility room to replace the soapy water I finally finished. The next day I found my patient walking around the ward completely cured! The head nurse had apparently chosen him to be my first patient and put him to bed so she could check off my first bed bath. In 2001 while I was hospitalized I was given a basin of water and some kind of liquid no-rinse soap that did not have to be washed off. I was told to bathe myself. This happened 60 years after my first encounter with a bed bath. It does take time for progress to progress! I had an IV in my arm, oxygen tube in my nose and was generally weak and discombobulated. There are other things I could say about my 2001 experience without back rubs, p.m. cares and employees dressed in colorful scrub suits with their level of expertise unrecognizable one from another. Sometimes it is difficult to recognize progress. I read somewhere "progress is not synonymous with change" or, one might add, not always. I can say this for the 2001 practices--there is less pneumonia from staying in bed too long!

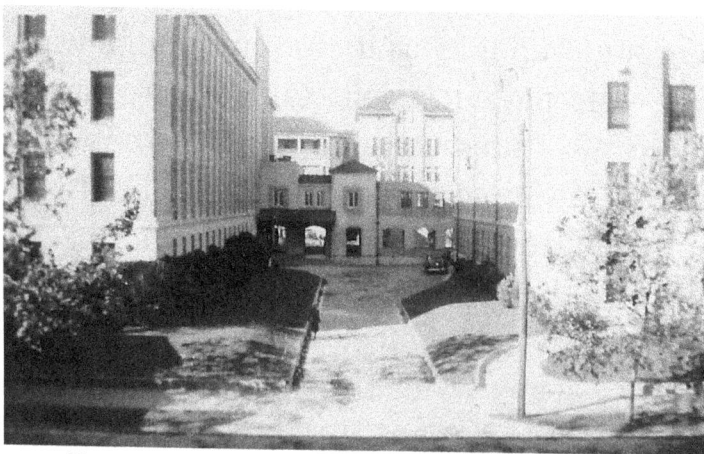

(Some of the buildings at John Sealy in 1941)

Back to 1941: At that time the pre-clinical students did all the direct patient care. Sometimes we had ten patients to bathe completely or help with a bath before we went to class at ten o'clock. Upper classmen gave medications, and someone was designated the treatment nurse. Senior students understudied the head nurse and at times replaced her. I always looked forward to the time when I would no longer have to give bed baths and could become a more lofty medication or treatment nurse. When I finally became an upper-classman new methods were inaugurated, and we were introduced to the "case method" in which one nurse did everything for a designated number of patients including the bed bath! This method is best for the patient in many ways. In 1999 during a hospitalization, when all sorts of people were doing all sorts of things for me, I talked with a soon to graduate, future RN about the care. She said they called it "fragmented nursing care." Personnel trained to various levels of expertise did their particular assigned task, and numerous people streamed through my room in the course of an eight-hour shift. I was surprised the word fragmented would be used, but I agree that was the kind of care I received. A fragment of care here and a fragment of care there with some fragments lost. The care was well named.

But back to Galveston and the 1940s: The Negro Hospital was built in 1937 and so was much more modern than the rest of the hospital. Segregation of black people from white people existed at this time. The hospital served women and children, as I remember. One day on one of the wards in the Negro Hospital I watched a resident doctor put into solution the first bottle of penicillin that I had seen. We had a woman patient with an advanced sinus infection in a private room. Some of the doctors doing research in the clinics had been allocated some penicillin, and a bottle of this new, fabulous drug was given to the resident for use for this patient. We all gathered around watching as he read the directions. He made the powder in the bottle into a solution and then gave a dose of the medication to the patient. We knew then we had entered a "new era." Our pharmacology teacher had explained to us that over time the bacteria treated with this drug would become resistant and then new drugs would be needed. However, we understood that for a time penicillin might cure the previously incurable. (I remember later, when I was an army nurse working a twelve hour shift for thirty days straight at Auburn General Hospital near McKinney, Texas, I gave penicillin every three hours to post-operative soldiers. At that time we withdrew individual doses from a small bottle of penicillin with a syringe and lined each syringe up on a tray with a corresponding medication card. By the end of the twelve hour shift I was almost "shell-shocked." Multiply that by thirty days, but that is really another story.)

I had come from a home in which we used some formality when addressing people. First name usage for adults was not in vogue generally, and definitely not in my background. When I arrived at the Negro Hospital Woman's Ward I addressed the patients using Mrs. or Miss preceding their last name only to be told by the head nurse that I should use their first names instead like Lizzie or Mary etc. I had much to learn. I considered the usage of first names too familiar. However, my background was West Texas not the Plantation South.

The Negro Hospital had one ward for Pediatrics. I remember three patients who were admitted at various times with strictures of the esophagus. Their mothers had used a solution of lye when they washed clothes and the children had mistaken it for water. The lye burned each of their esophagus causing strictures or worse. They received their nourishment, mixed in the Diet Kitchen, through a gastrostomy tube. They were such cute children and loved by all. One of the two little boys was having his esophagus stretched with a boogie in the operating room over a period of time, and much to his surgeon's sorrow one day the esophagus perforated accidentally and the child died. Another boy, about nine years old, had a dreadful case of psoriasis. His treatment consisted of oatmeal baths. I don't remember how frequently he received them.

After cooking the oatmeal we placed it in several layers of cheesecloth, and with the corners of the cheesecloth tied together the nurse applied the poultice to the child's body while he was in a bathtub filled with warm water. Many wonderful treatments as well as medications were yet to be discovered and used. May that statement be still true today whenever that today may be.

In 1926 the Medical School decided to create a Department of Neurology and Psychiatry. Dr. Titus H. Harris was a neurologist and took additional study in the field of Psychiatry. He headed the Department of Neurology and Psychiatry for thirty-six years. We received our psychiatric experience in the Psychiatric Hospital, a two story building, where all the patients, as I remember, were patients of Dr. Harris.

The first floor of the Psychiatric Hospital had two locked areas with one on either end of the building. Men were housed in one end and women in the other. I was one of the first students in our class to be rotated to this area and had not been introduced to psychiatric nursing. (Maybe they thought I was a natural for that area!) When I arrived the head nurse handed me a large procedure book for me to read and told me to let her know when I had finished reading it. Mostly, as I remember, the book described the physical facilities and stressed the fact certain doors always were to remain locked and the nurse in charge was responsible for the key. The patients under no circumstances were to have access to the key. After I told the head nurse I had finished the book we approached the locked door to the women's section. She unlocked the door. I proceeded through it; she followed behind and locked the door and put the key in her pocket. This was a pleasant looking unit of approximately 12 private rooms each opening off either side of the main corridor. At the end of the hall sat a grandmotherly type in a wheel chair silhouetted against the window looking much like the picture "Whistler's Mother." All of a sudden I heard a scream, "Go to hell and stay there!" A slender patient stepped from her door into the hall and called, "I wish you would stop that. You are driving me crazy!" Then a third patient appeared in her doorway and said "Why do you think you are here?" And that was my introduction to Dr. Harris' Psychiatric Hospital. Later the patient who had said "You are driving me crazy" told me she had been hospitalized because she got up in church and told the minister off, and she really didn't see why she should be put in the hospital for that. I questioned the head nurse who assured me there were more reasons for her admission than the one given by the patient.

Because all of the patients were private patients, we did not have access to their histories or work-ups. We had a general diagnosis to guide us. This was during World War II when many needs like sugar, shoes, gasoline were rationed, and you used coupons from your individual ration books to buy these items. I remember one patient, a young slightly built lady, diagnosed as a catatonic schizophrenic. She never spoke and only sat staring forlornly into space. The door to each room had a small window approximately twelve inches by six inches made so the patient could be observed if the door to the room was locked. This patient frequently stood on her side of the door with the window framing her eyes and blank expression. Someone told me the rationing system had overwhelmed her while she was trying to provide for her family. She had removed herself from the struggles of life. One night as I reported for night duty the nurse leaving told me the husband of this patient was going to arrive early in the morning and take her by car to the San Antonio State Hospital for further care. That night we had a special duty nurse with one of the patients. When she heard my patient's husband was coming to get his wife, the nurse took her cosmetics from her own purse and asked if she could fix up my patient's face so she would look pretty when her husband came. Why not, I thought. Her husband, very concerned and loving, arrived. He had covered the back seat of his car with blankets so she could lie down. She docilely crawled in and off they went to San Antonio. I don't remember whether we medicated her before she left.

At that time many of Dr. Harris' patients received shock therapy, either electric or insulin. Curare, a muscle relaxant, had begun to come into use in conjunction with the electric shock to keep the patient's bones from being broken during the patient's hard convulsions. The insulin shock patients were gathered in one room on low cots after they had been given their doses of insulin to produce the required shock. The insulin doses were much larger, of course, than those given to diabetic patients. It was difficult for me to give the large dosages after giving small doses of insulin to diabetic patients. I had to keep reminding myself I had checked the dosage, and the one I was giving was correct. Resident doctors gave orange juice and/or 50cc injections of glucose solution to bring the insulin shock patients out of shock if or when needed.

The second floor of the psychiatric hospital had private rooms. I remember one patient there who stalked about in his bathrobe and declared he was a Rosicrucian, an ancient order. I had never heard of Rosicrucians. A few of the patients were allowed passes to town for an evening out, I guess, to see if they could handle the outside world. Some were alcoholics.

A Woman's Building of four floors provided office space and space for medical and surgical units, a floor with private rooms, and obstetrics and gynecology. The top floor consisted of Obstetrics with the Nursery and Gynecology. One floor of this building had private rooms—perhaps no more than twelve. Here we honed our abilities to deal with a different type of patient than our ward patients. These patients had various conditions. I remember one patient in particular who had dreadful boils. Finally her doctor discovered the boils were self-inflicted by the patient injecting herself with milk. This was a quiet unit much different from our other experiences.

The Children's Hospital, built in 1937, provided care for many children under the Texas State Crippled Children program. The top floor included classrooms for the students who could get to the room. Also, a play area was available for the children where they could play or sit in the open air. These children had multiple surgeries requiring lengthy stays. To help keep them up with their school work an educational program provided classes for the school age children. This was considered quite "modern" and probably one of the few such programs in Texas, if not the only one, at that time.

As part of our clinical experience we spent several weeks in the Emergency Room staffed at times by one medical student and one student nurse. Occasionally we had some one brought in stabbed by a friend who would not prefer charges. We gave follow-up rabies shots over a period of time to patients who had come to the Emergency Room with their initial dog bite. Saturday evenings were the most active of all the week.

.

OFF- DUTY TIME

Our class of 69 students became friends and co-workers. We learned to know each other quite well. We depended upon each other at work. Also, we learned to respect the knowledge of the classmates in more advanced classes. Rules relaxed, and by the time I became a senior the custom of seniors entering elevators first was abandoned.

On December the 7th of 1941 while returning from church by bus someone getting onto the bus announced to all of us, "Pearl Harbor has been attacked!" With one voice we asked, "Where is Pearl Harbor?" We have all learned a great deal of geography since then. Television didn't appear until the 1950s so we relied on radio to get our news. As I mentioned before we would gather in the reception room of the Nurses' Residence to listen to President Franklin Roosevelt during his "fireside chats" consisting of information and comforting words over the radio. We would listen in hushed silence.

We had another hurricane in 1943 which caused much flooding in the Main Building particularly. By that time the medical students had either joined the

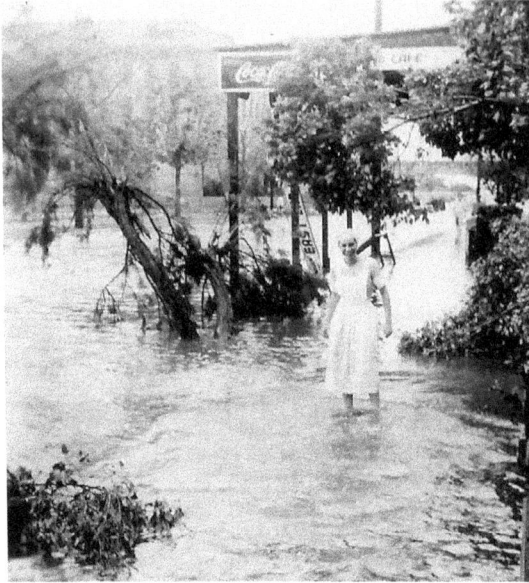

(A nursing student classmate wading in hurricane flood waters)

army or navy. The medical students, who were in the army, were brought to the hospital to mop out the basement. The Navy medical students faired better. Parts of Galveston are below sea level, and that basement was part of the below sea level area in Galveston. What a mess!

Each month I received twelve dollars from home with extra small amounts if direly needed. With this money I supplied what extra clothing I needed and incidentals with an occasional movie thrown in or a Mexican lunch at Market and 13th street. We actually needed very little since we were supplied uniforms and meals. However, it was relaxing to get away from the Medical Center for a few hours.

I would often take the trolley on Market Street to the library downtown on 25ᵗʰ Street and check out books and return on the trolley by way of Post Office Street. The Post Office was on 25ᵗʰ as well as the Depot and some of the piers. We were close enough to town to walk if we had time. We would go to the beach with friends and occasionally eat breakfast at a beach front restaurant where we would sit at a round table in the corner and watch the sea gulls wheel through the air and grab bread crumbs from friendly people.

When my brother Arthur was shipped overseas with the 90ᵗʰ Division he sent me a battered, tin suitcase holding his 8mm movie camera with film to be used and some cartoons for safe-keeping. Occasionally, I would get permission to show some of the films in the auditorium. One cartoon was THE BALOON MAN IN BALOONY LAND, and we would laugh heartily! My brother had taken pictures at the ranch showing trees being knocked down with a tractor. When I showed the film backward all the trees would stand back up in their place—an astonishing sight. Was life simpler then?

When I had a few days off after working night duty, I would take a taxi to the railroad station and catch the train from the depot in Galveston and go home to Uvalde. This was rather rare because someone would have to pick me up in Uvalde and take me to the ranch. Often, that was not possible. Gasoline and tires were both rationed. Also, the trains were very crowded carrying troops during this time.

There were a number of military bases nearby. Fort Crockett, Coast Guard I believe, was at the other end of the island. Many of our classmates dated and married soldiers from that base. Of course if a nurse married and the school authorities found out, she was immediately dismissed. (Smoking in the dormitory also was cause for dismissal). Camp Wallace near Alvin, and Ellington Field were nearby as well. There was an ancient and very tall wooden Roller Coaster near the beach in Galveston which when I rode it frightened me to death. I remember being so glad when we completed a round and I was ready to get off only to find we were planning on going around again!

The hospital commandeered our sugar coupons from our ration books. Food served in the cafeteria was generally good. I remember how we enjoyed dissolving an ice-cream bar into milk and imagining the concoction to be a milk shake. Two ice-cream bars made it taste even better. Sometimes we would sneak some sugar out of the Diet Kitchen and, with either bought or purloined cocoa, we would make fudge in an aluminum pan on an electric plate. We would stuff a towel against the bottom of our door so our house mother wouldn't notice our activity as this often occurred after curfew. She was a very nice person, and if she suspected anything she ignored what we were doing.

Our surroundings at the hospital were pleasant. Jack Tar Courts was on the way to Stewart Beach which was our nearest beach and frequent haunt. We often walked to the Ferry that connected Galveston and Point Bolivar. The Ferry carried cars and pedestrians for free. We would ride back and forth across the channel and watch the dolphins cavort in the water, listen to the sea gulls scream and then walk back to the dormitory. We would feel refreshed and renewed!

THE END

OR

PERHAPS, THE BEGINNING

My time spent in Galveston covered September 1941 to September 1944. At the completion of my three years of clinical experience my mother came for the final festivities. On my last day I worked my last few hours and found a friend to do the honors of partially tearing my old uniform to shreds as customarily done. Then dressed in my new white starched uniform with cap on my head complete with white hose and white shoes and accompanied by my mother we went to the hospital cafeteria for my last noon meal where we had the honor of the company of the Dean of the Nursing School, Miss Marjorie Bartholf, and my closest remaining friends.

My class of student nurses had participated earlier in a graduation ceremony in connection with the medical students, but each of the student nurses had to complete her three year stint, which varied, as I mentioned earlier, depending on vacations taken or time lost due to illness. It was a bit of a lonely time after watching some of my classmates finish and leave. I had wanted to stay and be a head nurse of a women's ward, but there were no openings for RNs at that time. Probably there were no funds available as well.

Later in the month in September I started working in the Operating Rooms at the Nix Hospital in San Antonio, Texas. With that position began a long and interesting journey.

Much has changed in the medical and nursing fields since 1944. At the end of World War II doctors returned from the army with refined skills honed by their many experiences. With the invention of plastic materials many new products replaced the rubber goods of our time. With the advent of public companies that produce medical supplies such as latex gloves and disposable equipment many of the tasks we had done were eliminated. Insurance companies now encourage early dismissal from hospitals. Times change, and the way we do things must change also; however, one may question whether progress is always synonymous with change.

EPILOGUE

When I have tried to tell people who at present are working in the nursing and medical professions about how it was when I was learning the Art of Nursing, they are incredulous. Washing, powdering, and autoclaving rubber gloves seems an impossible endeavor. They shudder at tales of hypodermaclysis with three inch long eighteen gauge needles. When I tell them about opening the first Recovery Room in the early 1950s for post-operative patients, they say they thought Recovery Rooms and Intensive Care Units had always existed. I suppose 60 plus years is "almost always," only I can remember how it was before we had such units. I hope when the current medical and nursing personnel tell how it used to be when they worked in the nursing or medical field their audience will be just as incredulous. The reaction to their tales will be proof new materials along with new knowledge have made new procedures possible.

Shakespeare wrote in "The Tempest" *(Act II, Scene I, lines 153-154)*

"whereof what's past is prologue, what to come is your and mine discharge."

How true! Each generation builds upon the previous generation's experience, knowledge and technology, and whatever today we are speaking about becomes the springboard for tomorrow.

I close with one final plea or hope. Equipment and treatments will always change, but one component in nursing care will always remain the same. The human patient, as a warm and feeling person, to whom we are giving all these wonderful treatments and procedures will always be present. Without his/her presence in the equation none of the other parts need to exist. The main goal is the care of the patient. Somehow the patient must not be forgotten during the rush to treat him. What a balancing act! The patient waiting in his bed for all the things that are being done to him appreciates the kind and gentle care given by a warm and feeling person who recognizes his needs as a fellow human-being. Minuscule things like being able to find the call-bell, being able to reach a glass of water, or get help to turn over may seem minor to hospital personnel but are monumental to the patient.

While writing these memoirs I couldn't resist making comments which may appear to be critical comparing the past with the present. I have been inactive from nursing since 1961, and my only experience with nursing care since then has been when I have been a patient or when I have observed care given to a loved one. However, for evaluation purposes, the vantage point of a patient may be the best way to view nursing care, and probably from that viewpoint the evaluation may be the harshest.

Let us hope in the rush and bustle of "today" there will always be that gentle someone following in the footsteps of Florence Nightingale, though she may be long forgotten, to do as Miss Nightingale laid down "the principle of nursing: careful observation and sensitivity to the patient's needs."

ADDENDUM

For the record the years I spent in the nursing profession included working at the Nix Hospital in San Antonio, Texas in the operating room, fourteen months in the Army Nurse Corps where I was an operating room nurse for most of the time, and as Assistant Director of Nurses at Santa Rosa Hospital in San Antonio, Texas after completing a Bachelor of Science Degree in Nursing Education from Incarnate Word College in San Antonio, Texas in 1947.

After I completed a Masters Degree in Nursing Education with a major in Hospital Administration and with minors in Public Health and Business Law from Catholic University in Washington D.C in 1950, the administrator of Santa Rosa Hospital in San Antonio, Texas rehired me, this time as Director of Nursing Service. I thoroughly enjoyed both of my times at Santa Rosa where I remained working even after I married.

My final employment in nursing included part-time night duty in the Intensive Care Unit and on medical surgical units at Santa Rosa and as a medication nurse at Lutheran General Hospital on Zarzamora Street in San Antonio, Texas. The hours of work in the nursing field were not friendly to a mother with children so in 1961 I changed careers and started teaching Special Education at South San High School, and in 1967 at Edison High School in San Antonio which was near home. My husband died in January of 1969 so I was very fortunate to have a job near home. While teaching in public schools, my vacations and working hours matched the vacations and school hours of my two children. I retired from public school teaching in 1982.

I have had the best of two very interesting careers and enjoyed both. More tales to tell!

www.ingramcontent.com/pod-product-compliance
Lightning Source LLC
Chambersburg PA
CBHW060640210326
41520CB00010B/1675